Essential Oils:
30+ Recipes For Beginners to Start With

The information herein is offered for informational purposes solely, and is universal as so. The presentation of the information is without contract or any type of guarantee assurance.

The trademarks that are used are without any consent, and the publication of the trademark is without permission or backing by the trademark owner. All trademarks and brands within this book are for clarifying purposes only and are the owned by the owners themselves, not affiliated with this document.

Table of content

Introduction

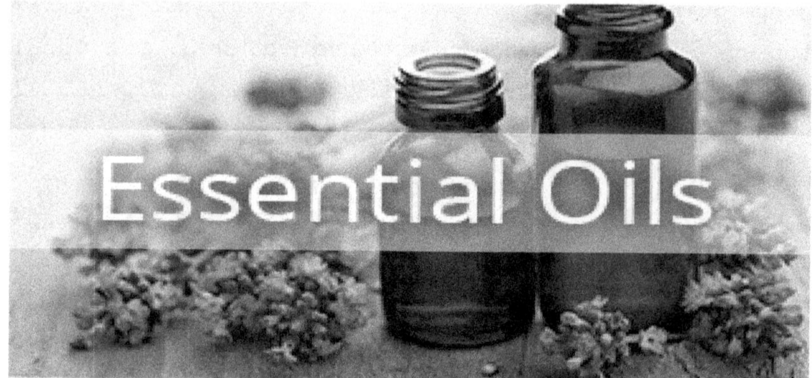

Essential oil is made from the distillation process of steam. Essential oils like many other natural products are among us for centuries. Person can get large benefits from them by consuming them in different ways like in cosmetics, diets or others. Essential oils are extracted from plants. Plants have it either internally or externally. If the essential oil is on the surface of the plant and you can feel it on your hands by just touching the plant, this means that it has external secretory structure. On the other hand, there are some plants that have to be plucked and cut in order to extract essential oils; such plants have internal secretory structure. They store essential oils internally. Basil, peppermint, marjoram and many others are essential oils common with plants having external secretory structures and Grapefruit, Cypress, Fir and many others are the essential oils found from the plants having internal secretory structures.

Essential oils are used in many ways but most common and beneficial ones are used through diffusion, taken in diets and applied on the surface of the skin. Because of its sweet, unique and soothing scent, essential oil can calm down the person, bring back the good memories and balance overall well-being.

In todays' world, due to poor diet, lack of physical exercise and extreme harmful toxins of the environment, person's body becomes unbalanced and energy levels are decreased. Essential oils can restore back the balance and manages your body weight.

Chapter 1 – Best Essential Oils for Stress & Tension

Essential oils are among us from the ancient times. It was used to treat the wounds of the soldiers in wars when there was scarcity of the medicine. The best part of the essential oils is that they are extracted from the roots of the plants, flowers or leaves of the plants. It is best to use essential oil that is pure and free from all kinds of chemicals. Essential oils are beneficial for curing many illnesses and help you find balance and cope with many stressful and anxious situations.

It has been proven through study conducted on some students that massaging with essential oils decreases the pain and depression and participants reported that aromatherapy massage, which includes use of essential oils, is more effective than the simple oil massage. So, next time you find yourself in a stressful state or you are anxious about something, try the essentials that are included in this chapter.

1. Lavender

Lavender oil is extracted from the Lavender flower and it is the most common oil which scents can soothe and calm the tensed person. Lavender has various components, 150 to be exact, they all interact with each other and help the person producing healing effect. Make sure to buy the lavender oil which is pure and of high quality, meaning it should have greater amounts of esters and low amount of cineol.

How to use:

All you need to do is to take few drops of lavender oil and apply it on the place it where there is any scar. Rub it gently till it gets absorbed. Keep on applying the oil till the area gets well.

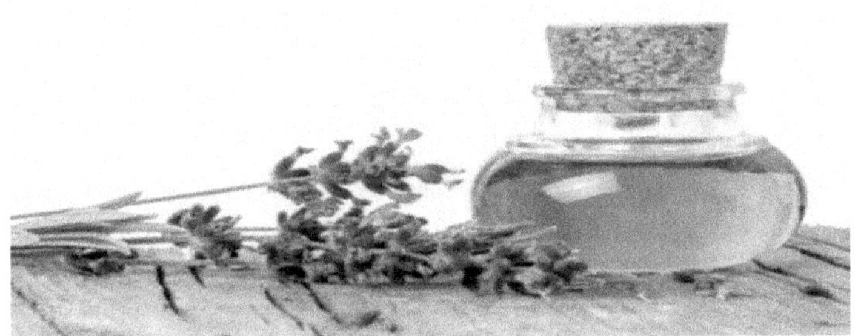

It is a known fact that the scent of Lavender oil gives inner peace to a person, helps the person to sleep and when it is inhaled, the brain's fast wave activity that is the main cause of anxiety is actually converted into the brain's alpha wave activity that is slower.

2. *Rose Geranium*

Rose Geranium has a sweet scent as roses mostly have. It has components that can balance the hormonal levels and relaxes the body; it also helps in making the person's mood in good state. Many people reported to feel relaxed and in light mood after smelling the scent of Rose Geranium. All this is because of the ability of this aroma to soothe the central nervous system and if ever you find yourself in a situation where you don't know how to cope with your tension and stress because of the workload or about your anxiety disorder, try sniffing this aroma. It has the ability to make you relaxed and take the pain away that is in your body.

How to use:

You can easily create massage oil by adding five to six drops of rose Geranium oil in one tablespoon of jojoba oil. Apply this oil on the place where you have pain. It will help to sooth pain. You can easily inhale the oil directly from the bottle for relaxation of the mind.

3. *Vetiver*

Vetiver Oil has an energy which is peaceful and grounding. It has been used to help the patients with trauma by making them self-aware and stabilized. It is the kind of tonic that helps nervous system to decrease the jitteriness and way too much sensitivity. It also helps in calming the person having panic attacks. It also has the effects of lowering the anxiety.

How to use:

Just add few drops of Vetiver oil in the water for bath. This will also give fragrance to the water and has cooling effect. This will allow to sooth your mind.

The other way to use is to add few drops of Vetiver oil with few drops of lavender oil and rose oil and apply it on the body. This will help you to relax yourself.

4. Ylang Ylang

Ylang Ylang has the most calming and soothing effects due to which it has been the most common and popular essential oil to treat depression and anxiety. It brings the cheerful person out in you who make you optimistic, happy and fearful. It can also help with the insomnia as it is a strong sedative.

It should be avoided by those who have low blood pressure. Study was conducted and it was observed that daily use of Ylang Ylang for four weeks reduced the stress and reduced the blood pressure of those with hypertension.

How to use:

Take eight drops of ylang ylang oil; 8 drops of lime oil, 6 drops of lavender oil 3 drops of clove oil. Mix them together. You can easily apply it to your body as massage oil. It will also give you relaxation and relieve your stress.

5. Bergamot

Bergamot has a very specific flower like taste and aroma and is usually found in earl grey tea. This essential oil has many benefits. It can help with insomnia and relaxes a person. It calms the person by increasing energy and decreases the agitation. Bergamot is known to balance and uplift the physical and emotional states of the body against stress.

For better results, it can be used with ginger, lavender and rosemary oils. It has a kind of aroma that calms the person by bringing the hypothalamus to its normal state of homeostasis. If you are in a lot of stress and tension, whatever might be the reason; this aroma might help you big time.

How to use:

Take 2 drops of ylang ylang with 1 drop of 1 drop of Bergamot oil. Apply this oil on the cotton ball. Inhale the vapor. It will give relaxation to your mind.

6. *Clary Sage*

This is another substance that when breathed in ought to be helpful for decreasing anxiety and nervousness. once there was a study conducted that included that breathing in clary sage with mixture of lavender, peppermint, and rosemary, these oils brought about less nervousness for the people taking an anxiety test. There have been a few studies conducted on the intake of clary sage and most have shown that it can help with stress and anxiety. It is not a complete cure for the anxiety disorder; however, it can ease and comfort the tensed body and thoughts momentarily. Few people also concluded that it might have properties as those of anti-depressants but this is questionable and has not been proven yet.

How to use:

Take 2 drops of clary sage oil and add 2 drops of peppermint oil with 3 drops of lavender oil. Massage it over your body. This will give relaxation to your body. This will help you to release the tension in your muscles.

7. *Sandalwood*

Sandalwood has a sweet, woodsy, outside sort aroma and can be exceptionally valuable in decreasing the tension and nervousness. There was a study conducted on sandalwood to see its effects on the illnesses that are terminal and it was observed that to decrease the general tension in these patients, sandalwood can be very beneficial. Furthermore, some have said that it works incredible to help with a sleeping disorder and also makes the person restful and calm. This aroma is originated from an evergreen tree and its oil has always been in the use of massage therapists in massage therapy which is from the heartwood. It also clears skin pigmentation.

How to use:

Take few drops of sandalwood and apply it on a cotton ball. Now inhale the fumes of the oil by breathing. This will get absorbed into your blood with the help of respiration and will help you to relax.

Chapter 2 – Essential Oil Blends for Weight Loss

While great nourishment and exercises are important steps toward getting more fit and keeping up a solid way of life, what people ignore on daily basis is that weight loss also includes attention to mental and physiological parts. Any individual who has attempted to shed more than a couple pounds realizes that there can be great difficulty in bringing the body and mind on same page, a forward and backward between one's genes, hormones, feelings, and the surroundings. Sadly for some people, just holding themselves away from food and doing regular exercise are not enough to lose some weight.

Essential oils are among us since the ancient times but have been used by the Chinese, roman, Greek and Indian people since the start for medicinal purposes. Nowadays, however, modern science is trying to conduct researches on how essential oils can be curative and how it can change the moods of the person and what others physiological properties it has.

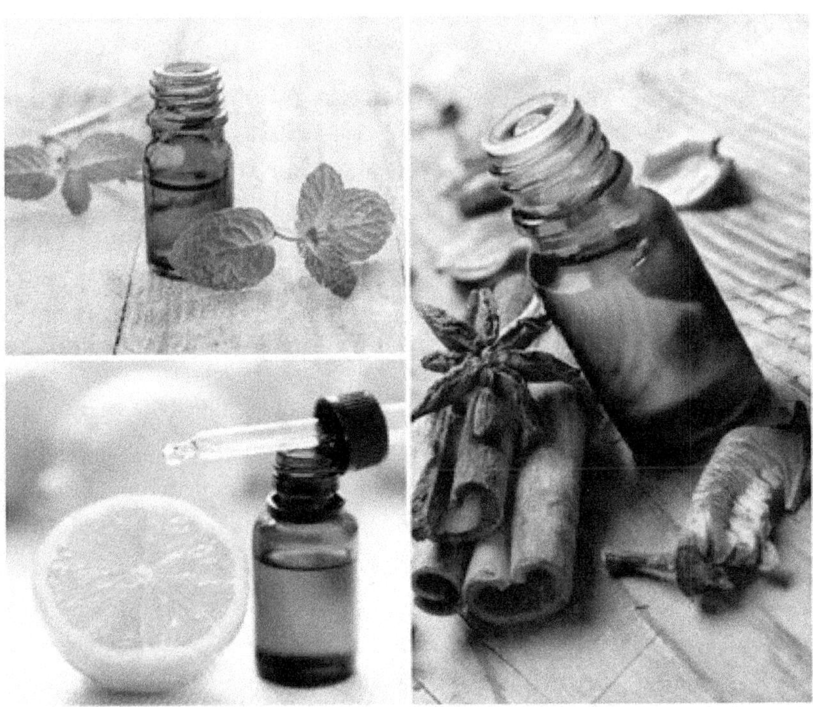

Before we go any further, it's important that you don't understand there is no easy way that you can lose weight. There's almost no scientific basis on the relationship between essential oils and weight reduction, and all things considered, proper diet and physical exercise are the best option for weight loss. But there are side benefits of essential oils and we will now put the light on how essential oils play their role in weight reduction. This chapter mainly focuses on the handful of essential oils that can actually help you with your weight loss.

8. *Lemon Essential Oil*

Lemon enhances energy, mood and give instant relief from pain and it suppresses gaining of weight. It contains the limonene that dissolves the fat. From the studies conducted, it has been found that lemon oil along with the grapefruit oil expanded lipolysis (that helps in breaking down the fats).

Lemon oil has the capability of treating the bad mood by reducing negative emotions. It likewise raises nor-epinephrine levels which is an anxiety hormone and neurotransmitter due to which a person is capable of deciding between the fight and flight in certain situations. Thus, the oxygen is expanded in the brain through nor-epinephrine so that the cognitive system can function better and increases heart rate and the flow of the blood due to which muscles work quicker.

Muscles' aches and strains may keep you from staying aware of your workout schedule, because of lemon oil you can get relief from pain and be more attentive.

How to use:

Take a glass of Luke warm water. Add 2 drops of lemon essential oil into it. Stir it well. Drink this water three times a day. This will help you to boost your metabolism and will promote weight loss.

9. *Grapefruit Essential Oil*

Grapefruit oil usually is used as antiseptic. It has a sweet and crisp aroma and it can restrain person's craving for food, has properties that can boost metabolism and enhances person's energy. Grapefruit contains a characteristic known as nootkatone which empowers a particular protein, AMPK to be exact, which helps control the energy levels of body and enhances metabolism. At the point when nootkatone is brought into the person's system, AMPK in the liver, muscles and brain's tissues chemical reactions. Due to studies conducted on the link between nootkatone and AMPK, it has been observed that it results in proper weight gain, loss of excess fat and improved physical activity.

One study was conducted on the rats, where they were presented with grapefruit oil three times a week so that they can smell it and with 15 minutes gap. They observed that rat's cravings decreased and its weight reduced. It is felt that limonene which is the grapefruit's essential part, creates lipolysis, which is the procedure through which fats are broken down and proteins are separated from them.

How to use:

Take a glass of water and add few drops of grapefruit oil into it. Diffuse this water in your office or working place. This will help you to decrease your appetite and craving. You can simply massage this oil on your chest or body whenever you have craving of food.

10. Peppermint

Peppermint has menthol due to which it is the most soothing and fresh and has calming effect. It increases the mental alertness and energy, brightens up the mood and helps in digestion while simultaneously decreases the appetite which makes it a good product for weight loss.

Because of its 70% menthol properties, peppermint has been used as a medicine for the indigestion for centuries. It has been found that peppermint is helpful in relaxing the muscles and when consumed with carway oil, it actually enhances the bile flow and eases the stomach muscles while lessening the bloating. All of this makes the nourishments to go through the body quickly. When compared with Ylang Ylang, it was observed that who inhaled the peppermint oil was more alert, was more relaxed and had enhanced memory function.

In a recent report it was mentioned that in a study the members who breathed in peppermint oil at regular intervals reported lower hunger levels and had taken altogether less calories. Hence, peppermint oil acts as an appetite suppressant.

How to use:

Take a cotton ball and dip it into peppermint oil. Now inhale the fumes of this oil. Practice this technique two times a day or whenever you have craving for food. This will help to suppress your appetite.

11. Fennel Essential Oil

This oil has been extracted from the seeds of fennel, and it is sweet and earthy. It helps in the weight loss by decreasing the appetite, improved digestion process and the person sleeps restfully.

Fennel has the hormone that directs the signals to brain regarding the daily wake-sleep cycle of a person. That hormone is known as Melatonin. Melatonin helps in the reduction of gaining weight by making the Beige fats rather than white fats. Beige fats are known to burn energy while white fats store energy.

Traditional folks when used to fast, they would take fennel seed so that their appetite can be suppressed.

How to use:

Take a cotton ball and dip it into fennel essential oil. Now inhale the fumes of this oil. Practice this technique two times a day or whenever you have craving for food. This will help to suppress your appetite.

12. Cardamom

It has been used by the traditional folks when they had to lose weight and the reason behind the fact that it can help in reducing the weight, might be that it has gastro-protective effects. Weight control starts from the stomach and ends with the stomach. It is not the fact that how much diet you take will determine your weight but how your stomach uses it. If there is any damage in the stomach or gut, it will waste even the proper diet as well. Cardamom oil is known to protect the stomach from ulcers and other damages. While using it, keep in mind that if you are internally using it then only one to two drops are more than enough.

How to use:

Take a glass of water. Add 2 to 3 drops of cardamom oil into it. Stir it well. Take this water once daily. It will help you to boost your metabolism and suppress your appetite.

13. Cumin

It hasn't been scientifically proven yet that consumption of cumin could help in weight loss, but it is a great herb overall, it helps in combatting the inflammation and diabetes. There has been studies conducted in which it has been observed that cumin consumption can affect the blood's sugar level of the body. Cumin is also an herb that is helpful in effective digestion system so it will be great if you add cumin oil to your weight loss blends. You can take it by adding it to the cooking or simply in diffuser as a part of blend.

How to use:

You can easily add cumin oil into any recipe that you eat. Another way is to drink a tablespoon of cumin seed oil as it is. This will help you to boost your metabolism and suppress your appetite. In this way you can loss your weight easily.

14. Ginger Oil

Ginger oil has the ability to reduce cravings for sugar and it has properties of anti-inflammation. It is important in a way that if you are trying to lose weight, it reduces inflammation of the body as well as it absorbs the important nutrients and it helps in digestion. Ginger has a gingerols compound that reduces the body inflammation by reducing the diseases that cause them in the intestine and also balances the vitamins and minerals in the body. If a person is consuming more than enough vitamins and proteins, they are helping their body's energy and they will lose weight.

How to use:

Take a glass of water and add few drops of ginger oil into it. Diffuse this water in your office or working place. This will help you to decrease your appetite and craving. You can simply massage this oil on your chest or body whenever you have craving of food.

Chapter 3 – Essential Oil Recipes for Skin Problems

Skin is the part of the body that is exposed most to the outer world and it is the largest part of the body as well. Due to the changes in the climatic conditions, skin gets affected and harmed in some cases when there are extreme weathers like in the monsoon seasons. The skin gets suffers from sweating, becomes dry or oily. In order to prevent that from happening, extreme care has to be taken of the skin. We have to adopt certain ways to protect the skin. Essential oils are used by many people to protect the skin from harmful conditions and it gives nice smell to the skin as well.

Body odors can also be cured by natural means, called essential oils instead of using artificial means like deodorants or perfume because these might include alcohol or other chemicals that probably will cause harm to the skin as it has been noted by many people that deodorants and perfumes if applied directly, produced skin discoloration. So, it is better to use the natural way to treat skin issues.

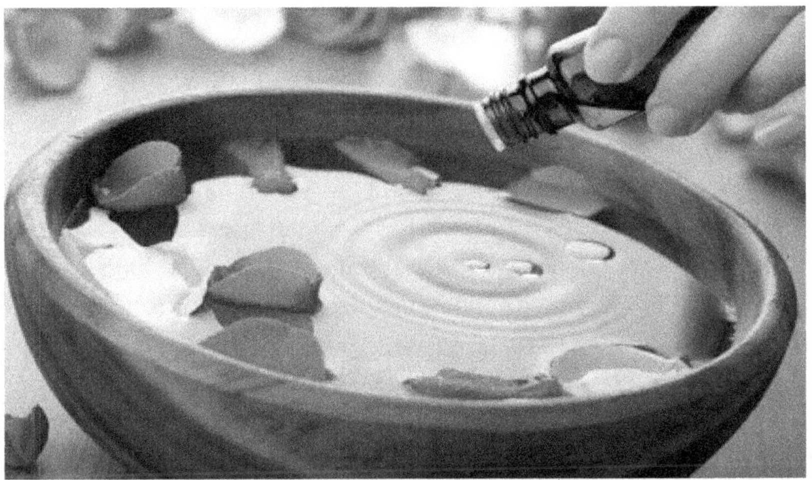

There are many essential oils available for skin problems, this chapter will focus on only few of them.

15. Neroli

Neroli oil might be a bit expensive but it has tremendous benefits for skin most importantly, it is beneficial for aging skin and stretch marks. It is also helpful in healing scars. Other than that, this essential oil can uplift the mood, comforts a person by calming him down and is also used during pregnancy. One thing should be kept in mind while using it is that it should be diluted.

How to use:

Add few drops of neroli oil in the lotion or cream which you use daily. Massage that cream or oil daily. It will help you to reduce marks on your body. Neroli has antibacterial properties that will help to reduce acne. Just apply oil directly on acne twice daily.

16. Myrrh

From the branches and woods of trees that are low grown, myrrh oil is extracted. It is an expensive tree and this oil shouldn't be used during pregnancy. For the dry skin it works best but is equally good for the oily skin as well. This oil is used for the conditions as dermatitis and is also good to heal scars and injuries. Myrrh has been used by many people with aging skin because it can reduce wrinkles very effectively as Myrrh oil contains anti-inflammatory properties and firms the skin, improving the skin tone and skin elasticity.

How to use:

Take few drops of Myrrh oil. Add few drops of Jojoba oil, almond oil and grapefruit oil. Mix them together and directly apply over any skin ailment. This will help you to get rid of that skin problem.

17. Frankincense

As this oil has the properties of anti-inflammatory and anti-bacterial, so it protects the skin from acne. This oil is like the natural toner that protects the skin from evening tone and pores. As it is cytophylactic, it protects the skin cells and even encourages the growth of new skin cells and due to this characteristic, Frankincense oil tightens the skin, improves wrinkles and heals the scars and soothes the skin that is dry.

How to use:

Take few drops of frankincense oil. Add few drops of Jojoba oil, almond oil and grapefruit oil. Mix them together and directly apply over any skin ailment. This will help you to get rid of that skin problem.

18. Rose Essential Oil

According to many researches, rose oil contains compounds like anti-microbial and anti-inflammatory due to which it has been considered as a great and most effective essential oil to reduce aging marks and dry skin. It also helps in refining the texture of the skin and also the tone of the skin. Other than that, it helps in managing certain conditions like dermatitis. According to one research, just inhaling the rose oil can diminish the skin's water loss.

How to use:

You can easily get rid of any blemishes with the help of rose oil. All you need to do is soak a cotton ball in the rose oil. Now apply this cotton on the blemish three times a day. If you want to get rid of acne you can do the same procedure by addition of coconut oil into it.

19. Tea Tree

Tree oil has been among the best solution to cure acne as it has anti-bacterial properties so it keeps the bacteria away from making any acne. It is the best source to produce oil on the skin due to which any skin breakage can be prevented or cured. Other than that, it is known for its ability to heal wounds. If you want to use tea tree oil to cure acne, put two to three drops of this oil on the cotton ball and put that cotton ball on the affected area, or it can be added to your daily face washing product, other than that you can use it via spray bottle by putting it in the spray bottle and spritzing it on the face whenever you want to.

How to use:

You can easily get rid of acne with the use of tea tree oil. Add two teaspoon of raw honey with five drops of tea tree oil. Rub this mixture on the face for 2 to 3 minutes. Leave it for 5 minutes and wash with plain water.

20. Juniper Berry

As the juniper berry oil has compounds of anti-bacteria and anti-microbial properties, it has been famous for the treatment of skin irritations and skin infections. It is a natural and home remedy, without side effects, for curing the acne and it also has properties that can lead to stress relief and detoxification due to which it protects the person in the situations where there is risk of getting or developing acne. You can use it by applying two to three drops directly to the area of acne or irritation, if you have a sensitive skin then you will have to dilute juniper berry oil with the coconut oil and then apply it.

How to use:

Take few drops of diluted juniper oil and add it with any carrier oil like almond oil, grapefruit oil or coconut oil. The ratio needs to be 1:1. Now apply it directly on the skin where there is any skin problem.

21. Patchouli

This particular essential oil is specifically very much beneficial for the aging skin
as it can reduce wrinkles and tightens the skin. What it does is, helps in producing new cells and their growth, smoothing the skin by smoothing the lines and
wrinkles. Patchouli oil has properties of anti-septic, anti-bacterial and anti-fungal, due to which it can help in making the skin conditions like dermatitis, psoria-
sis and eczema better.

How to use:

Take five to six drops of patchouli oil and rub it on the hand. Massage it on to the
place of skin inflammation. It will help to relive inflammation of that area.

22. Carrot Seed Oil

Carrot seed oil cures many of the skin problems but mainly the acne problem and
wrinkles. It repairs the skin and makes it more elastic by smoothing out the wrinkles. It works as detoxifier as well.

How to use:

Add few drops of carrot seed oil in the lotion or cream which you use daily. Massage that cream or oil daily. It will help you to reduce marks on your body. Carrot
seed oil has detoxification property as well. You can drink a teaspoon of this oil
to get rid of toxins of the body.

23. Rosehip Oil

This essential oil is specifically for the skin and has the qualities of smoothing the skin by repairing damaged skin, healing scars and reducing wrinkles and balancing the pH level of skin.

How to use:

Take few drops of rosehip oil and add it with any carrier oil like almond oil, grapefruit oil or coconut oil. The ratio needs to be 1:1. Now apply it directly on the skin where there is any skin problem.

24. Helichrysum Oil

This essential oil has been extracted from the flowers of the plants by the process of steam distillation. It has numerous benefits where there is skin concerned, it treats acne, heal scars and cuts and removes wrinkles.

How to use:

You can easily get rid of any blemishes with the help of Helichrysum oil. All you need to do is soak a cotton ball in the Helichrysum oil. Now apply this cotton on the blemish three times a day. If you want to get rid of acne you can do the same procedure by addition of coconut oil into it.

25. Pomegranate Seed Oil

It is a special essential oil in combating against the skin cancer. It has been used by traditional folks since ancient times because of its many benefits. Specifically, this oil is used for anti-aging, the dark color of pomegranate's oil helps in protecting the skin from sun's harmful rays if you put this oil before going out in the sun, on the skin.

How to use:

Add 40 drops Pomegranate Oil, 40 drops Rosehip Oil, 40 drops Rosehip Oil and 2 drops Rose Otto Essential Oil. Mix all the ingredients together in a bottle. Apply this oil daily. This will reduce skin problems. Use this oil within 6 months.

26. Jojoba Oil

Jojoba oil is not so famous but it is the best oil that contains many ingredients that are healthy like Vitamin E and Vitamin B complex, zinc and silicon. It helps in moisturizing the skin and hair and it also removes the excess oil on the skin and keeps the oil level balanced of the skin due to which if there is any acne, it will be reduced otherwise, it will prevent acne to rise.

How to use:

Take five to six drops of jojoba oil. Rub it on the hands and then massage on the face in circular direction. Do it for 5 minutes. Leave it there. Make it into practice before bed and in the morning.

27. Apricot Kernel Oil

Among the bests is the apricot kernel oil used to make skin healing blends. This oil contains too much omega 6 and it helps the skin to hydrate and nourish and it regenerates the skin collagen and cells so that wrinkles and fine lines can be reduced. It absorbs in the skin instantly so it is not greasy and is best for any kind of skin type. But most importantly, this oil is important for the skin healing and skin hydration.

How to use:

Take two teaspoon of apricot kernel oil. Add 3 to 4 drops of carrot oil, macadamia, avocado, olive oil and evening primrose oil. Add all these in a bottle and mix them well. This will act as a skin serum. Apply this serum twice daily.

Chapter 4 – Essential Oil Blends for Respiratory Problems

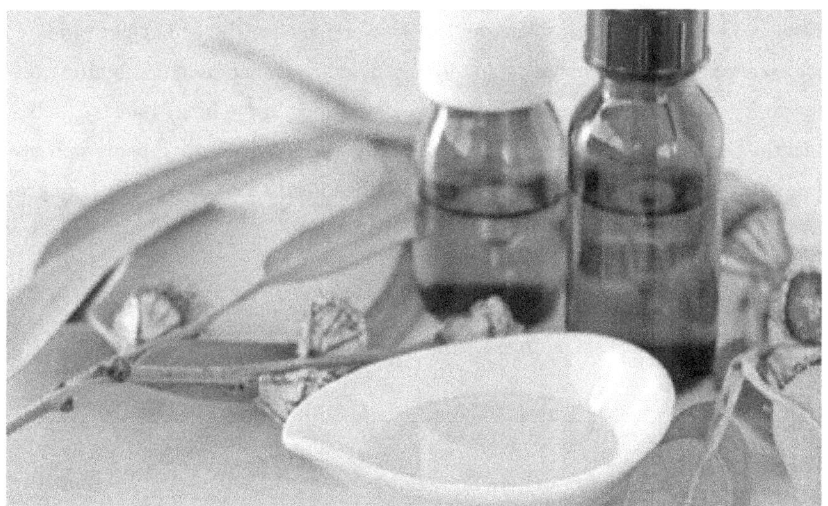

All respiratory issues arise because of the infections of numerous kinds. These infections attack the person particularly in winter season when the immune system is weak and is not able to fight against them all the time. Medications can for sure help us defeat most serious problems but leaving us with other many side effects and these medications mostly don't work in curing some simple illnesses like flu and cold. So, there is likewise another approach to enhance the health and make respiratory system stronger, subsiding the problems. That approach is the usage of proper essential oils.

These essential oils which are mentioned in this chapter and many others could be of great use of consumed in moderate amounts. If there are some serious issues, make sure to go to a doctor as they can be very dangerous. Essential oils soothe the lungs and heal many respiratory problems.

Nowadays, there are many viruses and bacteria out in the atmosphere due to which a person is exposed to them 24/7, hence, increasing the risk of getting different kinds of lungs diseases. There are some fluids in the lungs that try to protect the person to get an infection but as the amount of viruses and bacteria is rising, that fluid alone cannot face them all. Lungs need some help from us to protect them that is where essential oils can help us.

This chapter explains six main essential oils that can help protect the lungs.

28. Eucalyptus

There are two varieties of Eucalyptus essential oils; radiata and globulus. Both these varieties contain the compound called eucalyptol, due to which this oil has been famous for treating the colds. Apart from colds, eucalyptus oil is also essential for sore throats, cough and nasal congestion.

Both varieties of eucalyptus oil have properties of anti-bacterial and anti-fungal. Furthermore, they have anti-spasmodic and decongestant properties as well.

In order to use it, you can rub it directly to your chest area and the back upper area; this way the oil will be absorbed instantly and get to the lungs and from there to the bloodstream. Other way is to consume it through breathing in its steam by boiling it in water and draping towel over your head so that you can properly inhale the steam coming from that water.

How to use:

You can use eucalyptus by making steam bath. All you need to do is take a bowl of water and bring it to boil. Now add 2 tablespoon of eucalyptus oil into it. Now cover your head with a towel and putting face over the water. Take deep breath in this steam for 5 to 10 minutes.

29. Germ Killer Oil

Earlier, this essential oil blend was used to stop the plague and it has many benefits including the ability to boost immune system. It can replace many virus killing products like hand sanitizer, Lysol, bleach and other. It even helps in fighting the cancer. It can soothe throat irritation by gargling with the water containing two to four drops of germ killer oil. It also eases mouth sores.

How to use:

Take few drops of germ killer oil and rub it on the hands. Now apply it on the chest, massaging for 5 to 10 minutes. This will help relieve congestion.

30. Oregano Oil

Oregano oil has many benefits, it protects a person's body from many harmful foreign compounds and additionally, it has many psychological benefits. Since the ancient times, this oil has been used to treat upper respiratory problems, congestion and bronchitis. In order to use it, apply directly on the chest and upper back so that it can be absorbed by the skin to get into the lungs and into the bloodstream. Furthermore, this oil is useful in fighting off the infections.

How to use:

You can use oregano oil by making steam bath. All you need to do is take a bowl of water and bring it to boil. Now add 2 tablespoon of oregano oil into it. Now cover your head with a towel and putting face over the water. Take deep breath in this steam for 5 to 10 minutes. It will help relieve congestion and coughing.

31. Ravintsara

Ravintsara Essential oil is somewhat similar to eucalyptus oil and is extracted from the leaves of the same plant that gives away camphor oils. This essential oil is known to calm the person down and is helpful in emotional problems as well. It has been proven the best oil for lung problems as well as it contains eucalyptol just like the Eucalyptus oil. This essential oil is known to be beneficial for immune system and killing bacteria and other germs.

How to use:

5 drops Ravintsara oil, 10 drops Eucalyptus oil, 10 drops Melaleuca and 5 drops Thyme oil. Massage it all over the body except face. This will help relieve pneumonia.

32. Rosemary

There are many kinds of rosemary essential oils but for lungs, 1, 8 cineole chemotype is the most beneficial as it helps in boosting the immune system and protects the lungs from viruses and bacteria in a better way. It has the properties of antioxidant and anti-inflammatory. This particular essential oil can help in giving you relief from allergies, sore throats and many other conditions. It helps with asthma too.

How to use:

Take a cotton ball. Dip it into rosemary oil. Now inhale the vapors slowly. This will aid in relief of respiratory ailments.

33. Camphor

The essential oil high in camphor is yet another best essential oil for lung conditions as it contains antiseptic and antimicrobial properties. Due to its qualities, it can reduce infections and swellings and is helpful in giving instant relief from spasms by stimulating circulation. It is beneficial for many of the lungs conditions including congestion. Make sure to use this oil with great cautious and avoid consuming it with drugs as it can be narcotic itself.

How to use:

Take a cotton ball. Dip it into camphor oil. Now inhale the vapors slowly. This will aid in relief of respiratory ailments. This will also relieve the congestion of the nose.

Chapter 5 – Amazing Blends for Your Diffuser

Diffusing is basically a way to keep the air around you fresh and is used as a freshener. Essential oils used through diffusers helps in boosting the energy, improving the mood and change the mindset. It makes you focus on things and act as a stress reliever. All you have to do is put water in your diffuser and the essential oils, by turning it on it will poof out the aroma into the air.

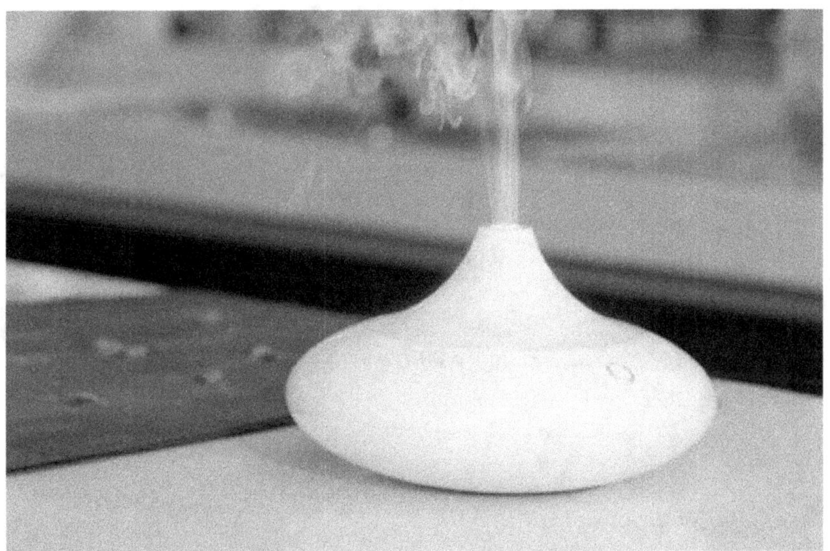

Following are the few amazing blends for your diffuser to start your day with:

To lift your brain and mindset, you can blend these together

- Peppermint oil: 3 drops

- Spearmint: 3 drops

- Wintergreen: 1 drop

To cope with stress during your day and have clear mind for challenging situations

- Lemon Oil: 4 drops

- En-R-Gee: 2 drops

In order to spend day with your family, try these by diffusing in the central area in the morning

- Lime: 3 drops

- Oola Family: 3 Drops

Essential Oil blends for More Energy

- You can blend earthy oils like frankincense and Ginger with herbs like peppermint, Rosemary and Basil. With these you can increase the levels of your energy.

- 4 drops of Peppermint and Wild Orange essential oil could also be combined when you have to work out.

Stress Relief Essential Oil Blends

- Lavender, Citrus, Floral oils, Clary Sage and citrus

- Roman chamomile-4 drops, Lavender-3 drops, Geranium- 2 drops, clary sage- 2 drops and a drop of Ylang Ylang

- 4 drops of Lavender, 2 drops of Orange, 2 drops of Cedar wood and a drop of Ylang Ylang

Essential oils for boosting Immunity

Blend these together to boost your immunity:

- 2 drops of each Peppermint, Lavender and Lemon essential oils. These are beneficial for clear breathing and healthy immune system

- A drop of Lime, Lemon, Rosemary, Peppermint and Eucalyptus essential oil in order to get rid of flu and other respiratory problems during winters

These were the basic blends you can use to have a refreshing experience. There are many other ways and you can even make your own by researching about the benefits of the oils you want to add.

Conclusion

Essential oils are of many kinds and consumption of essential oils is the natural way to soothe away many physiological as well as mental problems. Unlike other herbs and intakes, essential oils helps bringing the stress level down and makes the person feel more calmer and relaxed.

Essential oils like many other natural things are among since the ancient times and they are without any side effects, except when consumed in very large amounts. They have many benefits. In this book we have tried to cover the basic ones regarding the skin care, respiratory problems and weight loss. Many of the benefits have been scientifically proven; very few are yet left to be explored.

Essential oils can be consumed through different ways, applied directly and some are blended in diffusers. Their sweet and soothing aroma calms the mind and elevates the mood due to which person feels more energetic and positive towards spending the whole day either working or at home. For weight reduction, there are no scientific bases but through different essential oils, there could be decrease in appetite and improved digestion, due to which a person can reduce weight.

For skin problems, essential oils are very beneficial and almost every kind of skin problem can be cured via these precious oils. As they don't have any side effects so it is safe and easiest way to get rid of blemishes, stretch marks, scars, acne and whatnot? All in all, essential oil is the product of nature, extracted from the plants is very useful and could help you in day to day life.

FREE Bonus Reminder

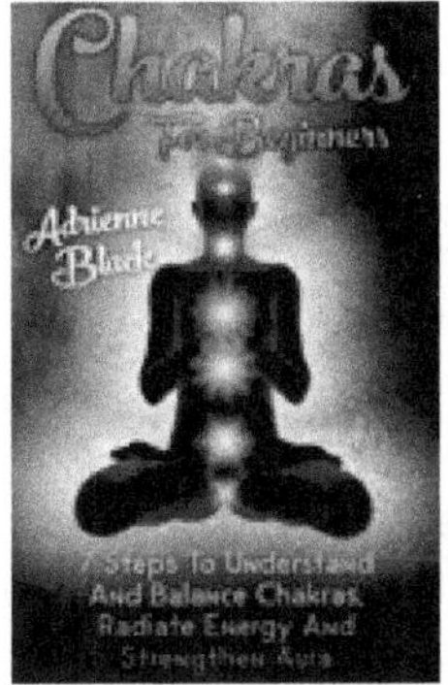

If you have not grabbed it yet, please go ahead and download your special bonus E book *"Chakras for Beginners. 7 Steps To Understand And Balance Chakras, Radiate Energy, And Strengthen Aura"*.

Simply Click the Button Below

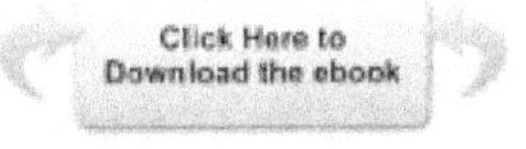

OR Go to This Page

http://lifehacksworld.com/free

BONUS #2: More Free & Discounted Books & Products

Do you want to receive more Free/Discounted Books or Products?

We have a mailing list where we send out our new Books or Products when they go free or with a discount on Amazon. Click on the link below to sign up for Free & Discount Book & Product Promotions.

=> Sign Up for Free & Discount Book & Product Promotions <=

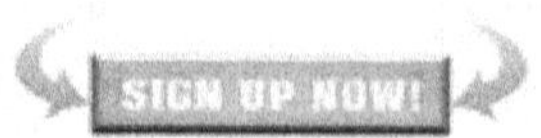

OR Go to this URL

http://zbit.ly/1WBb1Ek